To Diet Is To Fail

*The Powerful Way to Change Your Relationship
With Food and End Your Weight Loss Battle
Forever!*

Kevin Wichtendahl

"Dieting is wishful shrinking." -Author Unknown

Table of Contents

Dedication:

To my mother Elaine who has always been my biggest fan.

To my wife Teresa who lifts me up more than she will ever know.

To my children Brittney & Benjamin who have given me more joy in life than I will ever be able to give back.

Forward

The Beginning of the End

The great Yogi Berra once said that 50% of baseball is 90% mental. In the world of losing weight, 90% of weight loss is 99% mental. You may not realize it, but if you change the way you think and look at food, you will have a more dramatic effect on your waistline than if you were to work out 20 hours a day, seven days a week. This is not going to be some "psycho-babble" talk where we explore your childhood – but I am going to challenge you to look at your relationship with food.

This book was created to help you lose weight faster and more easily than you ever have before, but that is not the key to your long-term success. Forget about the fancy stats you have read that say x% of all people regain the weight in a certain amount of time. Instead, look at the popular NBC television show "The Biggest Loser" (yes, I love that show too). These people are given access to top-notch trainers, dieticians, doctors and are even offered cash to lose weight – and do they ever lose weight fast! But here is the sad part: did you know around 60% of them have gained nearly all of their weight back?

How could this be? I would think the sheer embarrassment would make me keep the weight off. Can you imagine walking down the street and having people recognize you from the show, giving you the "Oh my God – what happened to you?" look!

Bob, one of the trainers on the show, lost his cool with a contestant during an episode on the 2010 season. He felt she was too worried about winning the game, and yelled, "you will go home having learned nothing and gain your weight back!" I played that over and over again on my Tivo. If you are one of those people who like to put up inspirational messages on your refrigerator, you should start with that one!

If you have ever taken a diet pill, lost weight only to regain it – then you learned nothing.

If you have ever ordered pre-packaged food, lost weight only to regain it – then you learned nothing.

Diet pills, pre-packaged foods, and so many other ways to lose weight can offer short-term success, but do you really want to have to take a diet pill for the rest of your life? Of course you don't.

Imagine if you broke your arm. You would not listen to a doctor who told you to wear a cast for the rest of your life. The cast simply holds your arm in place while your body heals. When you have healed then you remove the cast. Think of this book the same way. It is my goal to try and heal you so you never have to take a diet pill or try the latest diet fad on the market.

My Story

I want to start off this book and the reason behind it with a story. It is a true story, but it is not about me – yet it led to me losing over one-third of my body weight. A couple of years ago, my wife and I attended a garden show. There was a line that had formed in front of one of the rooms where they were going to be demonstrating the latest break-through health device.

As we waited in line to get in, my wife engaged in a conversation with a rather large woman standing in front of her. Since we were standing in line for a health demonstration, the topic turned to excess weight and weight loss. The woman told my wife that she had undergone gastric bypass surgery over 18 months before. Due to her size, we were both surprised to hear that she had gone through this drastic surgery, and 18 months later, was still a very large woman.

Even though we did not say anything out loud to her, we must have been saying something with our eyes, because she immediately said, "Oh, I know I don't look so good now, but in the first year after the surgery I lost around 100 pounds – but in the last six months, I have gained most of it back."

My wife is a very sympathetic person, and expressed her sadness at this news and asked how it had happened. The woman explained that the surgery was very restrictive at first and also very good about keeping her from eating. The surgery also made her very sick whenever she overate, and this became very frustrating. But the good news (according to her), was that she had learned to "eat around it." It was then that she reached into her bag and pulled out a handful of bite-size candy bars. She said "I can pop these babies in my mouth, and I have no problem eating anymore!"

We were floored, shocked and appalled at the same time. I had looked into gastric bypass just a few months before this. I knew that the surgery this woman had gone through had cost her well over $20,000, and this estimate did not even take into account the pain, suffering and utter misery this woman had endured to have the surgery. And yet after going through all of this – this poor woman had "figured it out," and was now almost back to the weight she started at.

This incident bothered me for days and still does today. I went home and wrestled with this encounter and started comparing it to my personal history. I then started to think about all of the pounds I had lost, gained, lost again, and regained over the past 40 years. I had been on many diet plans like Atkins and pre-packaged meals that had been very successful for me. I had taken many different diet pills that help me lose a tremendous amount of weight. Yet, each and every time, I gained the weight back.

It was then that I started to really take notice of not only the thinner people around me, but also the heavier people around me. With the thinner people, I wanted to know how they conducted their eating lives differently than I had conducted my eating life up to this point. I believe to achieve any great goal in life, you need to model those that have already achieved it.

I decided to study those people around me who were struggling with weight issues, so that I could then study myself through my own eyes. You see, I believe that overeating is an affliction like so many others, where we get very good at lying to ourselves. We never believe we have a real problem. We tell ourselves that if we can just take a pill, go on the latest diet fad, or have surgery and lose the weight – we will never put the weight back on.

It was after studying other overweight people that I soon realized I was looking at myself. Let me tell you, that was a very sobering and frightening realization. Turns out, the fat guy going through the pizza buffet for the fifth time and telling himself he was going to start his diet tomorrow was me.

I finally realized that the only way to true health and lasting weight loss was to change my mental relationship with food. I needed to stop looking at food as a lover, a friend, and as a mind-altering drug. I needed to realize that food was simply a source of fuel for my body – nothing more and nothing less - and that it was I who had made food out to be so much more in my mind. I knew if I could change the way I thought and felt about food, the excess weight would come off.

And did it ever. In the next 18 months, I lost over 120 pounds, and it was truly the easiest thing I ever did. It was so easy because I had broken my relationship with food, and since that relationship was gone, so was the turmoil. The analogy I like to use is the one of the romantic break-up. When someone you love breaks up with you, it puts you in a tailspin, and there is nothing but pain and turmoil in your life. When you break up with someone though, you now have the power, and instead of turmoil, you actually feel relieved to have that individual out of your life.

I did not set out to write a book. In fact, it took coaxing from many others for me to actually do it. My struggle with weight has been a very personal

one, and I am sure it is no different than your own.
I can only hope and pray that what I have learned
will help you in the same way.

Retrain The Brain

For a lot of reasons, many that you do not realize, you are carrying more pounds than you want to. Why is it that you have always struggled with your weight but your best friend never has? Why is that we all know someone who can "eat anything they want" and never gain a single pound, while all you have to do is look at a piece of chocolate and you gain three pounds?

It is because they do not have a personal relationship with food. As soon as you de-personalize your relationship with food and just look at it as an object, your weight loss battle will be won!

We all started to develop our relationship with food as children. Food was used in a way that it should not have been used in your life (reward, punishment, scarcity, clean off your plate rules, don't waste it, etc). Why do you think obesity runs in the family? Some would have you believe it has to do with genetics and there are a lot of things that genetics, has an impact on blood pressure, heart disease and many other things. But do not think for a second that it is because of the genes you inherited from your great-grandmother that makes you eat three cheeseburgers for a meal.

For most of us overweight people we have tied the act of eating with one or many emotions. Perhaps you remember as a small child being in a setting surrounded by happy people. Maybe it was a birthday, a holiday or a family reunion. As a child you also noticed that these fun times there was usually an abundance of food around. Your subconscious mind was trained that people plus food equals fun!

Maybe as a child we noticed that when Dad came home in a really good mood he wanted to take Mom or even all of us out to dinner! Your subconscious mind was now being trained that family plus food equals security!

Then one day you were not having a good day as a kid. School was no fun; your best friend could not come over and play, or one of those other major problems we had as a child. Your mom saw that you were having a bad day so she gave you a really good carb and sugar-loaded snack to pick your mood up. And did it ever! Like an addict getting his first high, you were not sure what you ate made you feel so good – you just knew you wanted to experience it again and again. Now your subconscious just learned that a bad day plus food equals a MUCH better day.

Now our brain starts to tell us that food plus anything can equal fun, security or even make us feel better. Then your brain takes the next step and tells you if you are missing any of the other pieces like family, friends, excitement – just eat some food and everything will be all better. If I just described you then tell me what is the difference between you and the alcoholic who reaches for their next drink to deal with the same issues? Go back and replace "food plus anything else equals fun and makes me feel better" with "insert drug of choice here plus anything else equals fun and makes me feel better". If you have any experience with addicts in your life you will know there is no difference.

You need to stop thinking of food as a friend, a pick me up, or anything else other than food. **Food is just an object!**

Over the next couple of weeks you need to start to really observe people who are not overweight. Watch them when they eat and where they eat. I find the best place to do this is at fast food restaurants. Grab a booth in the back and watch healthy and non-healthy people order their food and then eat it. I know this may sound strange and I have gotten some strange looks from people but this little exercise will have an amazing effect.

Some of the things to note: Which group of people eat faster? Which group of people actually throws excess food away? Which group tends to eat alone?

After doing this a couple of times I actually got disgusted watching overweight people eat. I cannot describe this in a way that will give you the same impact of watching it for yourself. It was then that I realized "I am watching myself!" People who watch me eat are having the same feelings about me as I now have watching these people eat.

The next step to changing your relationship with food is another very simple exercise. Any time you are not eating at mealtime (breakfast, lunch or dinner) just ask yourself "what happened around me just before I started to eat this and what is my mood right now?"

Do this for about five days, and if you really want to change your relationship with food, actually journal it. When you review this after a few days you will start to notice a pattern. You will note how your mood at the time of eating is directly related to what you eat and the amount you eat. For me, I found out that I overate when I was either excited about something or down in the dumps about something. I also realized that I went for sweets when I was excited / happy and salty snacks when I needed a pick up.

Now comes the hard part. Now that you have identified the underlying issues you need to start fixing them. I know this can be easier said than done as some of these issues can run very deep. Often times we use food to help cope with self esteem issues, abandonment issues, relationships, financial situations and many more. It is very possible that the best thing to do is to seek professional guidance in dealing with these issues.

Regardless of how you choose to deal with these issues just ask yourself this – how did the bag of potato chips help you fix the relationship between you and your significant other? How did the gallon of ice cream make you feel better about being single or hating your boss?

Food did not help resolve any of these issues and it cannot because it is an object. Start to treat it as such and your life will better in more ways than you can even imagine.

Stay Out of the Bars

What is the difference between someone who over-eats at a buffet versus someone who drinks too much? I do not mean to trivialize the plight of anyone who struggles with alcohol, but I also do not appreciate anyone who has not struggled with over-eating trivializing the plight of an overeater. Remember you do not have to drink alcohol to survive, but you do have to eat food to live – so in this way, our struggle is actually harder.

Let's get this straight. My father suffered from alcoholism, as did my grandfather, and as did several of my aunts and uncles. So if anyone is in the place to make this comparison, I have earned the right. It is true that when I over-eat, I do not get behind the wheel of a car and put the lives of innocent people in danger.

Take a minute to look at the similarities between the plight of my father as an alcoholic and my plight as an over-eater:

- Neither of us felt we could stop once we started

- Both of us regretted how much we had drank/eaten the night before

- We were both triggered to over indulge by our emotions (happy, sad, depressed, bored, etc.)

- My father hoped none of his family or friends saw him when he was over-indulging. Nor did I.

- We were both ashamed we could not be like everyone else

So, follow the #1 rule that alcoholics are supposed to follow. Stay out of the bars! Or, in the world of over eating – stay out of the buffet lines and restaurants.

There is an old saying that says you cannot solve your problem until you admit you have a problem. My father could not go into the local bar and order a soda. The temptation was too great. I cannot go into a McDonald's and order a salad. It took me a long time to realize this. This has nothing to do with will power. Even if you could once, or even twice – you will eventually succumb to the temptation. So why even put yourself in that place to be tempted?

Yes, I had to change my life around a little bit, and in particular, my work schedule. I was in outside sales – a world where people like to be taken out, wined and dined. But here is the kicker: while I was losing over 120 pounds, I was also the top sales rep for my company for two years.

Speaking of alcohol – please do not make a habit of going out drinking while you are getting your weight under control. In my experience, drinking always leads to bad food choices.

To Diet is To Fail

You are not on a diet anymore. Follow the advice in this book, and you will never be on another diet again – ever. I hope that feels as good to read as it does to write.

Here is why the majority of people who lose a significant amount of weight gain it back – they have been brainwashed to think that in order to lose weight, they have to deprive themselves of what they love. This is a recipe for failure.

A personal trainer I know described her favorite foods as the foods that "talked to her." For her, salty snacks did nothing, but chocolate talked to her.

If you deprive yourself of what you love, you will fail. If you have been brain washed to believe that in order to lose weight, you need to deprive yourself of the foods that "talk to you," then you will surely gain the weight back.

In my opinion, this is the #1 reason that people from "The Biggest Loser" gain their weight back. They are never taught how to eat in the real world – dealing with the foods that "speak to them."

I love chocolate – I eat chocolate. I love a good steak – I eat steak. But when I do eat these foods, I do so in correct portion sizes (and not every day). We will cover both of these topics later, but rest assured that in order to fit into your favorite pair of jeans, you will not be giving up anything for the rest of your life.

Get It Out of the House

You cannot eat what you do not have. This may seem overly simple, but this could be one of the biggest ways you have sabotaged your past efforts. You may have the strongest desire to lose weight, but I guarantee that you will have a weak moment. You may have a sudden irresistible desire to eat some comfort food – so you do not want to make it easy to over eat. If it is not in the house, then you can not eat it. Sure, you can go to the store and buy some wonderful calories, but you have to drive or walk somewhere still to get it. And if it is after hours, then maybe the store is even closed. Regardless, if you force yourself to have to take the effort to go get the unnecessary calories, then during that time, you will have a chance to think it over and to really decide, "Do I want to eat this?"

So get up, go to your cupboards and hiding spots, and GET RID OF IT!

Now that you have gotten rid of it, do yourself a favor – do not buy anymore.

Does Taste Matter?

Quiz time: when was the last time you had a great meal, and what was it? If you can answer that one – then what was the time before that, and what was it?

If you are like most people, and if you are honest with yourself, then you will have a very tough time answering that question. I stumbled across this question when I was going through my struggles. My answer to that question was an awesome rib-eye steak that I had four months earlier at an anniversary meal. But wait, I thought – we overweight people eat because we love the taste of food, so why could I not even tell you what I had last week?

So, in theory, I could have eaten sawdust last week, and today, it would not have mattered. The good news is that you do not have to eat sawdust to lose weight. The better news is that the taste sensations and the memory of food tastes can be much less than you ever realized.

Here is an example from my own journey – I am a Diet Pepsi person. It seems that if you are a Diet Pepsi person then you are not a Diet Coke person and vice versa. I was out to lunch with a coworker at a place that only served Diet Coke, so I just ordered the regular Coke. During our lunch, the topic of dieting and weight loss came up. My coworker commented that I was drinking regular Coke on TOP of the un-healthy meal we were having. I explained to him my affection for Diet Pepsi and my dislike for Diet Coke.

He understood that, but noted that I had at least three large glasses (with free refills of course) of Coke during our meal. When I calculated it later, I realized I had just put over 700 worthless calories and 210 grams of unnecessary carbohydrates into my body!

I then decided that I would either start drinking whatever diet soda was available, or I would just drink water. The first couple of times it was not the greatest experience, but I got used to it. Now when

I go to a restaurant, my order is always for "diet whatever."

The same goes for light salad dressings, or light whatever. The problem is that we have convinced ourselves that we do not like the tastes of some things and will not eat them. What we have actually done is created a built-in excuse for not eating healthier. Trust me, I am well aware of the nasty tastes of some healthy foods, and I will not ever eat them again. Yet, there are many foods out there that once I got used to the tastes, they changed my life for the better. Expand your horizons and you will be amazed.

Important Side Note: did you know that the fastest way to gain weight is through liquids? Since there are no solids for your body to break down the nutrients, fat, calories, etc. – they absorb right into your body. This is why people who are severely malnourished are given liquids to get them back to health quickly. Stay away from unhealthy, non-filling liquids. If you were in my personal experience above, would you rather have 700 calories of soda or 700 calories of your favorite food?

Pass the Fiber

A study by Mayo Foundation for Medical Education[1] has shown that by just eating 30 grams of fiber every day, you will lose 10% of your body weight in a year.

This is with no changes to caloric intake and exercise level!

The reasons for this are simple:

1. Fibrous foods are more filling than non-fibrous foods.
2. Fiber keeps you regular. This is very important when you cut your caloric input, as you need to keep your body functioning at peak levels
3. Fiber is more difficult for your stomach to digest than other foods, so it actually increases your metabolism.

The bottom line is that when you are losing extra pounds, there is nothing stronger than to have fiber working for you. Instead of cutting your calories and having your body's metabolism shut down while you are feeling starved – fiber will immediately fill you up, and keep your metabolism up and burning calories.

Up until a couple of years ago, it was very hard to get 30+ grams of fiber in your diet. Not anymore! With the advent of fiber bars, such as Fiber One by General Mills, there is no excuse. They come in all sorts of flavors and have nine grams of fiber each. Eat one for breakfast, lunch, and with dinner, with eight ounces of liquid, and you will kill your appetite.

Bonus suggestion: if you are sweets lover, you may get a desire to indulge in a sweet treat now and then. As stated earlier, you should have thrown out all of the bad foods from your house and have plenty of fiber bars around. Go grab a Fiber One Cookies and Cream and enjoy it instead. You will satisfy your sweet tooth, and get your fiber in at the same time.

NOTE: Many people have commented about the gaseous and bloated feelings they get from fiber bars. Yes, that is a by-product of high fiber, but if you eat regularly for three to five days, your body will get used to it and the excess gas should stop. Just ask yourself this – would you rather put up with three to five days of feeling like a hot air balloon, or looking like one the rest of your life?

[1] November 19, 2009 - Mayo Foundation for Medical Education and Research (MFMER).

Sit Down!

If you are standing and eating – you are gaining weight! Period. Simple. End of story.

Why? There are two reasons. The first one is based on many years of reflection and also from watching other people. If you are standing and eating, that means you are doing at least two things at the same time – standing and eating. However, I would dare to say that you are actually doing even more than two things.

You are probably standing, eating and talking to someone. Or, you might be standing, eating and watching television. The point is, that out of the three activities you are doing, eating becomes a "mindless activity," and there is nothing good about eating being a mindless activity. What happens is that you are no longer concentrating on what you are eating, or even worse – how MUCH you are eating. So we always eat way too much when we do not think about it. In order to reduce the bad calories going in, you need to concentrate and think about what you are eating and if you are full.

The second reason actually comes from my doctor. I was sharing with her my rule on not standing and eating, and she said it was a brilliant rule but for a different reason. When we stand, we actually elongate our stomach. By doing so, we actually increase the amount of space for food to fit in and it takes much longer for us to feel full.

So do yourself a favor. Sit down, relax and enjoy your food. When you are done, concentrate on something else. If you are one of those who like to stand and talk at social functions, just put a bottle of water in your dominant hand instead.

Take a Probiotic

Have you ever taken an antibiotic? Then you need to take a Probiotic.

Have you even been on a diet before? Then you need to take a Probiotic.

What is a Probiotic? Let me give you the condensed, non-scientific version. You basically have little microorganisms that doctors call Gut Flora in your intestines. These microorganisms help break up the waste material that your body does not need and helps get it out.

Scientists have recently discovered two important things. The antibiotics we take for infections actually kill the Gut Flora. Putting your body on a crash/starvation diet can also destroy the Gut Flora balance in your body. When you are starving yourself, your body will start to shut down, and metabolism slows dramatically. Without food passing from your "intake to your outtake," the Gut Flora have nothing to feed on.

Doctors are now seeing a link between obesity, allergies and your immunity to certain diseases, to the lack of Gut Flora.

The good news is that it is very easy to correct this condition. You need to add a Probiotic to your diet. There are several easy ways to do this. There are several yogurts advertised that have Probiotics listed in the ingredients, and you can find these in any grocery store. My personal favorite is actually an incredibly small but powerful supplement called "The Pearl," which you can find listed at Amazon.com.

Do You Treat Your Car Like Your Body?

Next time you go fill your car up with gas, I want you to put in two more gallons than the tank will hold. So if your gas tank holds 10 gallons of gas, I want you to fill it up with 12 gallons. I am sure it will perform better...

You don't agree with me? Then why do you treat your body this way? It does not matter whether you drive a 1976 Pinto or a brand new Ferrari – cars do not perform better when you overfill their gas tanks. Your body is the same way – it will not perform better if you overfill it. You would never overfill your car because the gas would pour all over the ground. It would be a waste and a potential fire hazard. It is also a waste of money.

When you overfill your body with fuel (food), it does not perform better either. It is also a health hazard and a waste of money. The difference is that in the car analogy, you see the wasted fuel on the ground. With food, you see the wasted fuel around your body in the form of fat.

The next time you are hungry, ask yourself if your body really needs that fuel for peak performance.

Leave a Little, Lose a Little

Memorize this. Put it on sticky notes around your house. As mentioned earlier, the successful way to lose weight for the long term is to not deny yourself anything. However, to lose weight we do need to reduce what we are consuming.

Each time you are ready to eat anything – and I mean anything from a candy bar to a six-course meal - say to yourself before you begin, "leave a little, lose a little." Instead of eating the entire candy bar, throw away the last bite. Have the waiter take back your plate with food on it (and don't get it in a doggy bag). Throw away the last piece of pizza.

This will accomplish two things. First, if you eat less today – and by only a single bite than you did yesterday – you will lose weight.

Second, and more powerfully, is the mental strength and power you will feel by not eating all of it – especially for those people who were taught to clean their plates. The power to throw it away is one of the most powerful tools you need to successfully lose and maintain your weight loss.

Throw it in the Dead Sea

Do you pick at food in front of you after you are full? Give it the Dead Sea Treatment. That is, as soon as you have eaten enough, simply dump salt all over the food. Many people subconsciously pick at food in front of them while enjoying good conversation around the dinner table. Unfortunately, talking while eating distracts you from concentrating on eating. When you eat on auto-pilot, you eat too much. So next time you are done eating, simply grab the saltshaker and pour salt all over the leftovers. Don't have salt, or you really like salt? Easy – pour water all over it. Trust me, the next time you mindlessly pick at food you have poured salt and or water on, will be the last time!

Get on the Scale, Part I

You cannot manage what you do not measure; therefore, you need to get on the scale every day.

I know this is contrary to almost everything else you have ever heard about weighing yourself, but this could be a reason you are still struggling with your weight. The problem when you only weigh yourself once a week (or less), is that you cannot immediately reflect on what is causing the scale to go up or down.

If you get on the scale tomorrow and it says you have gained two pounds, you are able to instantly ask yourself "Okay, what exactly did I eat or do yesterday that caused the scale to go the wrong direction?" Conversely, when the scale goes down by two pounds, you can ask yourself the same thing, and do the exact same thing you did yesterday.

If you only weigh yourself once a week and the scale shows you gain weight, you have to remember EVERYTHING you ate and drank over the past week. And trust me on this one, you will never remember or be honest enough with yourself about what you ate over the last seven days down to the last bite.

Please note that I know there will be times when you do everything right, and your scale will either not move or will not move in the right direction. Women especially have this issue with water retention and their menstrual cycles. On the days where you know you have eaten less and the scale goes up – just remind yourself that this is a life-long change, and that your body will catch up.

As long as you are always honest with yourself, you will lose weight faster then ever before. You will also be amazed at what foods make the scale go the wrong way in a hurry.

Get on the Scale, Part II

Show me someone who is not getting on the scale, and I will show you someone who is gaining their weight back.

I have talked to and listened to hundreds of people who have lost a bunch of weight and then gained it back. 100% of them said that they stopped getting on the scale. Why is that?

Simple – they knew they were gaining the weight back, but decided to try and mentally fool themselves that they were not. To me, the scale should be your confessional. Good days, bad days, or any day – the scale will show you the exact reflection of what is going on in your life from a health perspective.

Bill Parcels, a great ex-NFL coach, once said, "You are what your record says you are." He said this in response to a reporter who was trying to ask him about some bad breaks in games (fumbles, penalties, etc.). His answer was that all of that does not matter because in the game of football, "You are what your record says you are."

In eating, you weigh what the scale says you weigh. It does not matter if it is your birthday or the holiday season or if you are on a cruise – you weigh what the scale says you weigh.

So if you really want to have real, long-term weight loss success, you need to change your lifestyle. Step one is to put a scale in a place where you have to walk by it every day, and to weigh yourself.

Go Back for Seconds, Thirds, Fourths, Whatever...

How many times have you put food on your plate, whether at a buffet or just when passing serving bowls around your table, and realized you took more food than you were hungry for?

More importantly, how many times has this happened and you have NOT eaten all of the food you took?

If you are like most overweight people, your answer to the first part of the question is much higher than your answer to the second part of the question. In fact, several people I have asked this question to did not even realize you could leave food on your plate.

There are several reasons people do this. Many will say that the reason they eat everything on their plate is that they were taught to do so by their parents. If this is your reasoning for doing this, than I would challenge you with this question – were your parents perfect, and did they do everything perfectly in bringing you up? Do you do everything today that they taught you? The answer is no, they were not perfect. In fact, if they were the perfect parents when it came to eating habits, you probably would not be struggling with your weight and your food choices today.

Regardless of the reason you feel compelled to eat everything on your plate, there is a very simple fix for this – stop taking so much food to begin with. Start by taking half of the food you normally do. Eat it slowly. When you are done – repeat the process.

By following this really simple way of eating, you will be amazed by how much less food you eat.

Water, Water, Everywhere – The Secret of Hollywood

I had the opportunity to see a roundtable discussion of a group of A-list actors and actresses discuss a film they had done. There was a table of eight of them on stage; it included the stars of the film as well as directors and producers. About 30 minutes into it, I noticed something. Each one of them had a bottle of water in front of them and at least two more bottles of water by their feet.

Why was this? Did they all have the same high sodium meal beforehand? Was the room hot and they needed to cool off?

No. The reason they all were drinking water, is that they know that drinking water is key to not eating. And when you are not eating, you are not gaining weight. Here is what they have learned about drinking water:

- Many overeaters also have an "oral fixation." That is the need to have their hands and mouths doing something all of the time (this is why many overweight people also struggle with smoking, chewing nails, etc.) Having a bottle of water in your hands at all times will satisfy this subconscious need.

- Are you thirsty or hungry? Did you know most people have a hard time telling the difference? When in doubt, drink some water instead of eating something.

- It fills you up. Find a book on the human anatomy, and you will see that the stomach has a finite size. Yes, yours could be smaller or bigger than others, and yes, you can make your stomach larger by eating more continually – but the bottom line is that your stomach can only hold so much. If you fill it with water, then there will not be room for anything else *(please note this is an example – drinking only water can and will lead to serious health issues).*

Do Not "Inhale It" – Make Sure You "Enjoy It"

Ask 100 overweight people why they eat so much, and 100 of them will give you the same answer: "Because I love the taste of food."

Really? Then why do you eat it so fast? Apply this same logic to other areas of your life, and see how much sense it makes:

- When you have sex, do you get it over as quickly as possible, or do you want to enjoy every second of it?
- When you go on vacation, do you want it to last for five minutes, and then go back to work?
- When you are sitting down to read a new novel by your favorite author, do you want the book to be two pages long?

Before you dismiss these as stupid analogies, really ask yourself this: why do you eat so fast and take such big bites? Remember, you are eating so much food because you love the taste, and want to have more of what you love.

I came to this realization when I was traveling recently. A gentleman who had stopped by a burger stand in the airport got on the plane and brought the burger on board with him. I was seated in the next aisle across from him, so I could witness this without appearing rude. This burger was a monster – you name it, and the burger had it on there. It probably cost close to $10.

He started eating it and began to take the biggest bites imaginable. His mouth was completely full with each bite. At the end, which was about six bites worth, he commented to the gentleman next to him that it was an "awesome burger!" How would he have known? If it was a truly "awesome burger", why not enjoy every last bite and make the taste last as long as possible? The flight was two hours long, so it was not like he was rushed in any way. By the looks of him, he was not starving in any way either.

There are three key things you need to take away from this story:

- It is a well-known fact that your stomach needs approximately 30 minutes after starting eating, to tell your brain that it is full. This is why when you overeat you feel so miserable AFTER you have overeaten, rather than while you are eating. If you are jamming food into your stomach as quickly as possible, by the time your brain says you are full, you will have done some major caloric damage to your body.

- Do you want to look like this guy did when he was eating? Start watching others eat. The perfect place for this is a mall. Just sit down at a table with a newspaper and quietly observe how people eat. Start to emulate how the thinner people eat, and you will soon be one yourself.

- Enjoy it. Savor the flavor. If you are overweight because you truly love the taste of food, than do yourself a favor and really enjoy it.

Guard The Perimeter

I have a friend who is a business consultant and coach. He is one of the most disciplined individuals I have ever met. Yet, even though he is the king of discipline, he knows his limits.

Every Sunday night he orders the same caesar salad to go from the same restaurant. Every time he places the order, he tells them to not include the free loaf of garlic bread. And every week, they include the free loaf of garlic bread. When he gets home, he walks over to the dumpster and throws the bread away.

Why? Because he knows that if he allows the bread into the perimeter of his house, then he will eat it. Even though this man is the king of discipline, he knows his limitations and you also need to know yours. There is no reason to tempt yourself when you can avoid the temptation completely. Do not bring the leftovers home. If someone gives you a gift of food – give it to someone else.

Stay away from those deals where if you buy X, they will throw in free breadsticks or upgrade your order to the next size. Yes, it will cost you a couple bucks more, but you will not have the temptation to deal with. Any extra money you think you will be saving will be converted in extra pounds.

Only you know what your true limitations are. You need to be honest with yourself enough to know that if there is extra food in the house it is like a little voice in the back of your head that is calling you to eat it.

I cannot tell you how many times I have gone to the cupboard looking for something sweet and or salty to eat. Since I guard my perimeter (our house) very closely, that type of food does not exist in our home. There are times when this can annoy me. When I do not find the food I am craving I have the choice to go find something else or I could jump in the car and head to town to grab something. I have yet to grab my keys to head to the store. Yet, if the unhealthy food had been in the house – I surely would have eaten it. By keeping it out of the house, it is no longer a temptation.

The Power to Throw Food Away

Several times throughout this book, we have discussed throwing food away or destroying it. To many of you this is a foreign practice and perhaps even borders on criminal action. You need to prove to yourself that you are in control of your life and that food is not. The best way to do this both consciously and subconsciously is to throw it away. When you throw perfectly good food away, you will discover a power within you that you did not know you have always had. Each time you do this, the power increases along with your sense of pride.

Take One Extra Step

To most of us, we find exercise neither easy nor fun, but it is very simple to begin to see it in this way. First of all, do not wake up tomorrow and commit yourself to working out 30 minutes a day for the rest of your life. To do so is to set yourself up for failure. Instead, start out with this simple goal: Take one more step today than you did yesterday. That's it. They say the road to success starts with one step. The road to losing weight and getting into shape starts with one extra step.

When you go to work or shopping, park just one spot further away from the front door than you did last time. Do you normally take the elevator at work? Go to the stairs, walk up two steps, walk down and then get on the elevator. Tomorrow walk up three steps, walk down and get on the elevator. Each day, simply add one and repeat. Before no time at all, you will have walked off many pounds and have created a very healthy and simple exercise routine that did not cost you a dime.

Stop Lying to Yourself

Does this sound familiar: "I can't believe I did not lose weight yesterday – I had NOTHING to eat," or, "I am going to order a big dinner tonight because I have had NOTHING to eat all day."

Liar.

I don't mean to offend, but you and I have used these statements when talking to ourselves and we know this is a lie. I know very few people outside of third world countries who truly go all day without eating anything. Whether you are sticking your finger in frosting, having a small bite of chocolate, or just some leftovers – you are eating. Overeating and eating junk is one thing - lying to yourself about it is another.

In order to be truly successful in losing weight, you need to start being honest with yourself. You are responsible for every pound you have put on. You are responsible for everything you put in your mouth.

Prove it To Yourself

Do this simple exercise: grab a pencil and a small notebook you can stick in your pocket. Every time your hand goes to your mouth and you swallow, write it ALL down. From coffee (include the cream and sugar), to soda, to gum – write it down. At the end of three days, go over every line and see how much "nothing to eat" really adds up to.

A friend of mine purchased one of those workout DVDs she saw on television. It called for her to work out for 20 minutes a day, six days a week. It also had an eating plan with it as well. She did the routine for three months and saw almost zero results on the scale. Since she had three months invested into a better body, she was determined to get the results she wanted. She took a small notebook and carried it with her wherever she went. Anytime that ANYTHING went into her mouth, she just wrote it down. She did not go and look up the calories each item had – she just wrote it down. At the end of the week, she sat down and reviewed her notes. In under a minute, she knew exactly why the scale was not moving. She had no idea she was eating as much as she was and as often as she was. She simply made a mental note of the areas she was succumbing to food temptations and corrected them. You see, the mind is so much more powerful than we can ever appreciate. Write it down; read it; tie emotion to it and whenever that situation occurs, your mind will remind you of the emotion you originally felt.

She dropped over 30 pounds in a little over a month. She also learned a very important lesson: people tend to UNDERESTIMATE the calories they take in and OVERESTIMATE the calories they burn!

Stop Lying to Strangers

I was recently on a trip and noticed a gentleman ordering french fries at a buffet line. When he got the fries, he asked the server for some more and stated, "A buddy of mine and I are sharing them." The server just smiled and gave him twice as many fries.

I did not follow the man back to his table to see if he was lying or not, but I can tell you this – A) he was overweight, and B) if he was not lying this time, I believe in the past he has lied about food before. If not, why would he be so quick in front of complete strangers to try and justify his request with the "sharing with a buddy" statement? It was all you can eat.

Have you ever ordered food in a drive-through, for delivery or anywhere else, and tried to make total strangers believe you were not going to eat it all yourself? Based on my personal experience, and those of most overweight people I know, I would bet that you have, too. The only reason you do this is that you are embarrassed about the amount of food you are about to consume, and you feel guilty for doing so. From now on, commit to yourself that you will never lie to others about food quantities.

This will allow you to accomplish two important things:

- If you follow the earlier rule on going back for seconds, you should never have to use this excuse in the first place, and you will give your body time to tell you if you are really still hungry

- You will begin to emulate those who are successful at maintaining their proper body weight. Those people never lie to others or get embarrassed about their food choices.

What is Your Trigger Food?

We all have them and chances are you already know what it is. You know, the food that you eat, that once it hits your lips your appetite explodes – and no matter what you do, you cannot seem to get enough of it. In other words – what food calls out your name like the seductress it is?

For some it is bread, for others it is potato chips, and for others, it can be sweets like chocolate. The food that the majority of people will answer with is a carbohydrate. This is actually the theory behind the popular, and somewhat successful diet referred to as Atkins.

The problem with Atkins is that it has labeled all carbohydrates as trigger foods, and that is simply not correct. For example I can eat one piece of bread and couldn't care less for any more, but open a bag a chips and hold me back! There was a commercial on years ago that summed it up the best, "I bet you can't eat just one!" I lost that bet every time.

What you need to realize is that there is something within your trigger food that sets off the intense craving for more. There is an ingredient in your trigger food that affects your mood and general feeling of well-being. It may also cause an emotional stimulus. For example, when you are very sad, the caffeine in chocolate perks you up – or, when you are excited and happy, the white flour in bread intensifies that feeling even more.

The next step after you have identified your trigger food is to avoid it like the plague. Do not buy it, do not have it around the house, and do not eat it. Yes, you can save for very special occasions a couple times of year, but otherwise, you should do whatever possible to avoid your trigger food.

Get Right Back on the Wagon

Imagine you are late for work and that you have to break the speed limit to get there on time. Then, a stoplight changes to red just before you get to the light. You do not see anyone coming through the intersection, so you run the red light. Thankfully, you are safe, but even with running the red light and breaking the speed limit, you still arrive at work a couple minutes late. Question for you – do you now run every red light and break every speed limit for the rest of the day? I am sure the answer is no.

Yet, you do the exact same thing when you overeat. Regardless of your willpower, there probably will be a day or two in which you eat more than you should, or something that is not healthy for you. When this happens, why is it that you say to yourself, "Well, I blew my diet for eating that for breakfast, so I might as well just blow it for the whole day." That makes about as much sense as the red light example from above.

Treat each meal and each time you put something in your mouth as a separate event. What happened this morning does not dictate what you will eat for lunch.

We all make mistakes and poor choices from time to time. It is OK to forgiving yourself. Just tell yourself that you forgive yourself for your poor eating choice, and get right back on your plan.

The Picture Trick

Have you ever found a picture of yourself when you were at an ideal weight, and placed that picture on your refrigerator to help you lose weight? How did that work for you? It did not work for me at all. Then, I met with a professional corporate trainer/physiologist on a totally unrelated topic, and we began discussing weight loss issues and failures of mine. What he told me blew me away.

He told me about studies that show the human mind will do more out of fear than out of hope. A little deep, I know, but let me give you an analogy. If you were timed in two different races – running the exact same distance, which of the following would you run faster toward:

       a. Running toward a bowl of ice cream (or favorite food)

       b. Running from a bee that was trying to sting you

99% of us would have run from the bee faster! Or, consider this:

a. Running toward a big pile of cash

b. Running from an angry bear

Research shows the answer is b again. While I am sure they did not test this out on actual bears, this analogy can still be used to make the point that fear is a stronger motivator than desire. So, how does this help you lose weight?

Go find a picture of someone of the same gender and skin color who is substantially bigger than you. Put that on your refrigerator. Better yet, take that picture and cut out a picture of your face and put it over that image's face. Now, put that on every refrigerator or area of temptation in your life. I guarantee that your mind will do everything in its power to make sure you do not get that big. The problem with the picture of you skinny, is that it does not put fear in your mind, and therefore, it is not that powerful. Just try this method for a couple of days, and you will be amazed at the power of it.

When you reach your goal weight, then replace the picture with a picture of you at your heaviest. You will not go back to that weight again.

The Exercise Trap

As mentioned several times before, I lost over 120 pounds and did not exercise for a single minute. That is not some sales pitch, but the God's honest truth. Why? Because I knew I would fall into the same exercise trap I had fallen for so many times before, and if you have ever exercised to try and lose weight, I am sure you have unknowingly fallen into the same trap.

The trap: I worked out this morning, so I can have the doughnut. I am going to work out again tomorrow, so I can order the french fries instead of the vegetables. To remove the trap, you can remove the excuse. Whether you like it or not, the main reason you have gained weight is because of everything you have eaten, not because of a lack of exercise. Trying to commit yourself to changing your eating lifestyle, and committing yourself to exercising six days a week is a commitment to failure.

Here is how powerful this trap is. Now that I have reached my goal weight, I am able to do things like exercising more easily. I joined the local YMCA so that I can get in better cardio shape and tone up some areas of my body. Even after all of the weight loss and everything I have learned – I still hear the voice when I am eating, saying, "You worked out today really hard – you deserve the ice cream cone. We will work it off tomorrow." I have to tell my inner voice to shut up and stick to my plan. This trap is so powerful that if I cannot contain it, I will quit my exercise program.

One Victory a Day

Nothing builds confidence like success. In the game of football, it is very important that the quarterback is the most confident player on the field. In order to build confidence in a young quarterback, the coaches always start out games by calling very short and easy pass plays. They do this to instill a sense of confidence in a young player, so that they are more confident when it comes to the big plays.

You need to do the same thing. When you are reviewing your day and how well you did, you need to look for the small victories, not where you think you made mistakes. For example, on a recent vacation trip, we all stopped at a gift shop. Everyone else grabbed an unhealthy snack. I did not. Later on that evening, we stopped at a restaurant and I think I ended up eating more than I should have.

When I looked back at the day, I focused on the stop at the gift shop. That was a huge victory, and is something that to this day I have built on. I know that I am capable of saying no to food, and I will continue to do so.

Look for your victories every day, regardless of how small, and you will soon be winning all of your battles with temptation.

The Compliments That Can Destroy

By now, you are seeing the weight come off like never before. People around you are now noticing you and complimenting you. A word of warning – do not listen to them!

Everyone loves a compliment, especially about losing weight. However, you will find that these compliments instill a false sense of success and security. There is a saying in sports about the danger of reading your own headlines, because you may actually start to believe them. The same goes for weight loss.

When people get compliments, they tend to get over-confident in their own abilities. They start to think that they have this weight loss thing down, and that they can simply turn it on or off as they need to. Worse yet, you start to see that you have won this battle, and begin to think you can stop. To reuse an overused cliché: this is not a destination, but a journey. Since we are not denying ourselves anything, and simply eating in moderation – we can and will eat this way for the rest of our lives.

So do yourself a favor. Take the compliment, say thank you and do not give it a second thought.

The Friends and Loved Ones That Can Destroy

Do you think your overweight friends and/or spouse wants you to succeed at this? The real answer will shock you.

Once when I was somewhere in the middle of my weight-loss journey, my wife was in another part of the house visiting with her mother. Her mother made the comment about me losing weight rapidly and so effortlessly. I was in the next room and overheard this conversation:

Mother-in-law: "You have to be really happy with him and his weight loss."
Wife: "I am – he is really doing a great job."
Mother-in-law: "Are you really happy about it?"
Wife: "NO! I think it sucks that he can lose weight and I can not!"

Was I angry? No – I was a little shocked, but I was happy that she was being honest. Later that evening, we discussed it in detail. My mother-in-law knew to ask the question because she has struggled with her weight in her later years, and knew what it was like to have a spouse lose weight. She also knew her daughter.

If you have any overweight friends you can be assured they are thinking the same thing. What is worse for them is when you start going places together and people start commenting about your weight loss in front of them. It will get very tiresome for them in a hurry. I have actually had to apologize to my kids for others who just went on and on about my weight loss.

If you have ever been on the other side of this, I am sure you know what this feels like. Regardless of your intentions, it can be very hard not to get bitter and jealous over this issue.

The best way to handle this is to simply be prepared for it. Know that not everyone will be thrilled for your success. It is sad to say that you may actually lose friends over this, and then you will need to decide what is really important in your life. I hope you will choose your health over any selfish, insecure friendships.

The Friends and Loved Ones That Can Sabotage

As discussed earlier, not all of your friends and loved ones are going to be thrilled with your success. Neither you nor they might consciously recognize this, but these same people will also be the ones that will try and knock you off of your new lifestyle and back into theirs. You may not believe this to be true, but I have seen it countless times in other relationships, and even in my own.

It can start with the following comment "How much weight are you going to lose?" Translation – they are not comfortable with their own size, and your continued weight loss is going to make them even more uncomfortable, so STOP NOW!

Then your favorite food starts showing up around the house. When you ask them why they are buying your trigger foods, they tell you it is only for a special occasion, or it was on sale, or because you have done so well, it is a special treat.

These are all methods in which those around us are actually trying to sabotage our efforts. Depending on the person it can be subconscious, or even conscious. The usual suspects are spouses, parents, children and friends. Just have your guard up and pay attention for this, and you will be amazed at the saboteurs lurking in the weeds.

Here is what I do. When they bring home the food I do not want in the house, I take it with me, like I may actually eat it. Then, when they are not paying attention – I destroy it, either down the drain or in the garbage. This way, I avoid the confrontation about their actual intentions, and I exercise my power to throw away food.

Pick Your Best Friend Wisely

I always advise couples to read this book together, and if you are not married, then to go through it with a close friend. Your best friend needs to be your voice of reason in times of weakness, and vice versa.

Let's say you have had a lousy day at work, or a tough day with the kids. When you say to your best friend, "I have had a tough day. Let's head to our old favorite restaurant for some serious carbs!" At this point, you do not need your friend to say, "Great – whose car are we taking?"

Instead, you need your friend or spouse to say, "That is an option, but let's go for a walk instead to get rid of some of that stress." You need someone to kindly and lovingly remind you of your goal, and what is really important. You need support – not an enabler. Make sure your loved ones around you know that you are trying to change your life for the better, and ask them for supportive strength when you are not at your strongest.

Just Try

A national news show recently did a story on weight loss. Over the last 10 years they had done three major stories on weight loss and different methods people had used to lose weight. These three methods were:

- No carbohydrate plan
- Major calorie reduction
- Eating only non-processed foods

The news program decided to go back, review all of the stories and do a follow up on the participants.

Guess which one was the most effective? They all were.

Guess which one had the most people gain their weight back after a year or more? They all did. Not everyone who participated gained all of their weight back, but each weight loss approach had participants who had gained all of their weight back.

At the end of the report, the reporter said that in reviewing the people who had participated in these programs he thought the main difference was those that were successful "just tried" and maybe that was the key to weight loss.

Just Try..

Every day is not going to be easy. Every day is not going to be filled with success. You can give up and then what? Back to where you started yet again.

They say that to make any relationship in your life work you need to work it at everyday. If you are married there is no time when you can cross the finish line and say "Well, I got this thing taken care of." If you do, then your next stop will be visiting a good divorce attorney.

There are no alcoholics or drug addicts that will wake up tomorrow and declare to the world that they are now cured.

Maintaining and controlling your weight is no different. This is a journey, not a destination. By making small and simple changes to your life this journey can be very easy and enjoyable.

I wish you the best of success on this new journey. You can do it. Just try.

Made in the USA
Charleston, SC
06 March 2011